OSTEOARTHRITIS

INTO ALL IT TAKES TO HEAL

OSTEOATHRITIS

DR. A. RAMOS

Contents

INTRODUCTION

Osteoarthritis, often known as OA, is a common degenerative joint disease that mostly affects cartilage, which is the tissue that covers the ends of bones in a joint and provides protection. The progressive degeneration of cartilage in this long-term illness causes joint discomfort, stiffness, and decreased suppleness. While osteoarthritis can affect every joint in the body, it is more common in weight-bearing joints including the spine, hips, and knees.

Bones may rub against one another when cartilage deteriorates, resulting in pain, edema, and the development of bone spurs. Osteoarthritis has multiple etiological variables, including genetic, mechanical, and environmental aspects. Although older folks are more likely to experience it, younger people may also be affected, particularly if they have joint injuries or other risk factors.

Osteoarthritis is managed with a mix of exercise, drugs, lifestyle changes, and occasionally surgical procedures to reduce symptoms and enhance joint function. Effective management solutions attempt to improve the quality of life for people who have osteoarthritis, despite the fact that there is no known cure. For persons who have osteoarthritis and the medical professionals who support them, it is essential to comprehend the origins, symptoms, and available treatments.

CHAPTER ONE

What Osteoarthritis Is Not

The smooth, protective tissue that coats the ends of bones in a joint, cartilage, gradually deteriorates in osteoarthritis (OA), a degenerative joint disease. Cartilage facilitates painless, seamless joint movement by acting as a cushion. Osteoarthritis is characterized by gradual cartilage degradation that results in joint discomfort, stiffness, and loss of suppleness.

Important Osteoarthritis Features:

Cartilage Degeneration: The main feature of osteoarthritis (OA) is the gradual degeneration of cartilage in the afflicted joint. Aging, wear and use on the joints, and genetic factors can all contribute to this breakdown.

Joint Stiffness and Pain: When cartilage deteriorates, bones may rub against one another, resulting in joint stiffness, pain, and swelling. This pain is frequently more noticeable right before or right after movement.

Diminished Joint Flexibility: Bone spur formation and cartilage loss can cause a reduction in joint flexibility. People who have osteoarthritis (OA) may find it difficult to bend, squat, or carry out other tasks that call for a broad range of motion.

Osteophytes, or Bone Spurs: One of the most common characteristics of osteoarthritis (OA) is the development of osteophytes. These bony protrusions may form around the bounds of the injured joint.

Joint Effusion: Osteoarthritis (OA) may result in the build-up of fluid in the joint, which can cause swelling and pain.

Osteoarthritis can affect any joint, although it most frequently affects weight-bearing joints like the spine, hips, and knees. The hands and fingers are two other joints that are frequently impacted.

Gradual Onset: The course of osteoarthritis usually takes a while to develop. Although it is frequently linked to aging, joint traumas, obesity, and genetic factors can also cause it.

Osteoarthritis is associated with several risk factors, such as age, genetics, obesity, joint injury, and repetitive joint stress jobs or activities.

Osteoarthritis is managed with a combination of pain medications, exercise, lifestyle changes, and, in certain situations, surgical interventions. Although osteoarthritis cannot be cured, those who suffer from this degenerative joint disease can greatly enhance their quality of life with early detection and appropriate treatment.

Reasons and Danger Elements

There are several variables that contribute to the development of osteoarthritis (OA), including environmental and genetic factors. Numerous variables contribute to the beginning and progression of osteoarthritis, even if its precise etiology is not entirely understood. The following are some typical osteoarthritis causes and risk factors:

1. Age:

Aging is more frequently linked to osteoarthritis. As people age, they are more likely to develop osteoarthritis (OA), which is more common in those over 65.

2. Genetics:

There is a genetic component to osteoarthritis susceptibility. Certain people may be genetically predisposed to developing osteoarthritis (OA), particularly if there is a family history of the ailment.

3. Joint Damage:

Osteoarthritis in the affected joint is more likely to develop in cases where the joint has already sustained trauma, such as fractures or tears in ligaments. The deterioration of cartilage may be accelerated by joint trauma.

4. Overweight:

Osteoarthritis is significantly more likely in those who are overweight, especially in weight-bearing joints like the knees and hips. Because obesity puts more mechanical strain on joints, cartilage deterioration results.

5. Repetitive Stress and Overuse of Joints:

Osteoarthritis can occur as a result of some jobs or hobbies that require repetitive joint movements or put an undue amount of stress on particular joints. Workers, athletes, and those in physically demanding occupations can be more vulnerable.

6. Misalignment of the Joints:

Damage to cartilage can result from structural abnormalities or joint misalignments, which can be acquired later in life or present from birth. These conditions can cause uneven pressure on the joint surfaces.

7. Gender

Women are more likely than men to develop osteoarthritis, especially after menopause. It's possible that hormonal changes contribute to the higher incidence of OA in women.

8. Hormonal Elements:

Changes in hormones, including those that happen during menopause, can have an impact on osteoarthritis development. Changes in joint tissues have been related to estrogen levels.

9. Combined Unstability:

Osteoarthritis may occur as a result of conditions that create joint instability, such as ligament injuries or certain joint illnesses.

10. Factors related to metabolism:

Diabetes and several types of crystal deposition diseases are examples of metabolic disorders that may raise the risk of osteoarthritis.

11. Genetics:

Genetic and family history can influence a person's propensity to develop osteoarthritis. Variations in certain genes may have an impact on the composition and integrity of joint tissues.

It is possible to identify those who are more likely to develop osteoarthritis and to use early detection and preventive actions by having a thorough understanding of these causes and risk factors. Although there are certain risk factors that cannot be changed, joint protection techniques, weight control, and lifestyle changes can significantly lessen the effects of osteoarthritis.

Indications

Osteoarthritis (OA) can cause a wide range of symptoms, with individual differences in symptom intensity. The following are typical signs of osteoarthritis:

Joint Pain:

Osteoarthritis is characterized by persistent discomfort in the afflicted joint. The pain may get greater during or after activity and is frequently described as aching or throbbing.

Hardness:

stiffness in the afflicted joint, particularly in the morning or after extended periods of inactivity. Stretching and light movement may help the stiffness.

Joint Inflammation:

swelling and inflammation in the injured joint, which causes the joint to enlarge. Most of the time, the swelling is restricted to the joint and may be heated.

Decreased Range of Motion

Reduced range of motion and limited flexibility in the afflicted joint. Osteoarthritis patients may find it difficult to bend, squat, or extend their joints entirely.

Collaborative Crepitus:

the joint's internal grinding, grating, or crackling sound when moving. The noise, called crepitus, may be felt or heard by the person.

Sensitivity:

To the touch, the afflicted joint may feel sensitive, particularly in the vicinity of the joint borders.

Pain Associated with Bearing Weight:

Pain that gets worse as you walk or stand and is more common in weight-bearing joints like the knees and hips.

Pain Management while Resting:

pain temporarily relieved by resting or by reducing joint activity. Resting the afflicted joint can help osteoarthritis sufferers feel less uncomfortable.

Combined Deformities:

In more severe instances, osteoarthritis can result in the creation of bone spurs or alignment abnormalities in the joints.

Anguish due to Weather Shifts:

Some people with osteoarthritis claim that cold temperatures or low-pressure systems cause their joints to hurt or stiffen more.

It's crucial to remember that osteoarthritis symptoms can worsen with time and that not everyone who has the condition will have them all. Furthermore, comparable symptoms may be presented by other joint disorders or inflammatory arthritis, emphasizing the significance of a precise diagnosis made by a medical specialist.

Obtaining a medical evaluation is crucial for a correct diagnosis and the creation of a suitable treatment plan for people who think they may have osteoarthritis or who have ongoing joint pain. The quality of life for those with osteoarthritis can be greatly enhanced by early intervention and lifestyle changes.

Identification and Medical Assessment

Osteoarthritis (OA) diagnosis is made using a combination of physical examination, medical history evaluation, and, occasionally, imaging investigations. The following are the main elements of osteoarthritis diagnosis and medical evaluation:

Health Background:

The first step for healthcare professionals is to get a thorough medical history, which includes details about the exact joints afflicted, the type of pain experienced, when the symptoms first appeared, and any triggers for the symptoms.

Evaluation of Symptoms:

An assessment of common osteoarthritis symptoms, including stiffness, swelling, discomfort in the joints, and decreased range of motion. Making an appropriate diagnosis depends critically on the location and nature of the symptoms.

Physical Assessment:

A comprehensive physical assessment is performed to evaluate the impacted joints. This involves measuring joint discomfort, checking for swelling or inflammation, and gauging joint flexibility. In addition, the medical professional might look for joint abnormalities and movement-related cracking.

Joint Imaging

To see the afflicted joints, imaging tests like X-rays and, occasionally, computed tomography (CT) or magnetic resonance imaging (MRI) may be requested. X-rays can show changes in bone density typical of osteoarthritis, bone spurs present, and narrowing of the joint spaces.

CHAPTER TWO

Blood Examinations:

In contrast to several other types of arthritis, osteoarthritis is usually not linked to notable alterations in blood indicators. To rule out other forms of arthritis, like rheumatoid arthritis, blood tests are typically carried out.

Analysis of Synovial Fluid:

After a joint aspiration, the synovial fluid the fluid inside the joint may be examined to check for inflammation and rule out other forms of arthritis.

Evaluation of the Functional Impact:

Assessing how osteoarthritis affects a person's everyday activities and functionality is crucial. This could entail evaluating one's mobility, capacity for carrying out particular tasks, and general impact on quality of life.

Standards for the Diagnosis:

Medical professionals may base their diagnosis of osteoarthritis on recognized criteria, such as those set forth by the American College of Rheumatology, which take into account radiological and clinical findings.

It's crucial to remember that osteoarthritis is frequently diagnosed clinically, taking into account a patient's history of symptoms, physical examination findings, and imaging data.

Osteoarthritis cannot be definitively diagnosed with a laboratory test; instead, the condition is generally diagnosed by ruling out other possible causes of joint discomfort.

Following a diagnosis, the patient and the healthcare team can collaborate to create a customized care plan that may involve medication administration, lifestyle changes, pain management techniques, exercise regimens, and, in certain situations, lifestyle changes. It might be advised to schedule routine follow-up visits in order to track the development of symptoms and modify the treatment strategy as necessary.

A multimodal strategy is used to address osteoarthritis (OA) with the goals of symptom relief, improved joint function, and overall quality of life enhancement. Among the osteoarthritis treatment options are:

Changes in Lifestyle:

Weight control: It's important to keep a healthy weight, particularly for joints that carry weight. Losing weight can ease symptoms and lessen joint tension.

Exercise: Low-impact activities that build muscles, ease discomfort, and increase joint flexibility include swimming, cycling, and walking. Customized workout regimens may benefit from physical therapy.

Pain Control:

Over-the-Counter Pain Relievers: Ibuprofen and naproxen, two examples of nonsteroidal anti-inflammatory medications (NSAIDs), can help lessen pain and inflammation.

Topical Analgesics: Localized pain relief can be achieved by using creams, gels, or patches containing analgesic drugs such as diclofenac or capsaicin.

For people who are unable to take NSAIDs, acetaminophen is a painkiller that may be suggested.

Prescription Drugs:

Analgesics: Due to possible hazards and side effects, the use of prescription-strength painkillers, such as opioids, is usually restricted. However, they may be explored in specific instances.

Intra-Articular Corticosteroid Injections: By injecting corticosteroids straight into the injured joint, pain and inflammation may be momentarily reduced.

Physical Medicine:

Exercise regimens created by physical therapists can strengthen muscles, increase joint flexibility, and improve joint function overall. They might also instruct people in cooperative protection methods.

Helping Tools:

Orthotic shoe inserts, canes, and braces are examples of supportive equipment that can aid increase stability and lessen joint tension.

Injections of joint hyaluronic acid:

Some people may benefit from intra-articular hyaluronic acid injections to relieve discomfort and give their joints extra lubrication.

Surgical Procedures:

Surgical alternatives such arthroscopy, joint realignment techniques, or joint replacement surgery may be explored when conservative approaches fail.

Regenerative Health Care:

The possibility of novel therapies including mesenchymal stem cell therapy and platelet-rich plasma (PRP) injections to promote tissue repair and lower inflammation is being investigated.

Learning and Self-Control:

Educating people about osteoarthritis, how to manage it, and self-care techniques encourages them to take an active role in their care. It's crucial to learn joint protection strategies and make lifestyle changes.

Support and Guidance:

It might be difficult to manage osteoarthritis' effects on daily living and chronic pain. Support groups and counseling could be advantageous for mental health.

The intensity of the symptoms, the joints that are impacted, and the patient's general health are taken into account while creating treatment regimens. It is essential to follow up with medical professionals on a regular basis to discuss any changes in symptoms or the course of the illness, modify treatment plans, and assess the efficacy of actions. In order to optimize outcomes and improve quality of life, successful therapy of osteoarthritis frequently entails collaboration between medical professionals and those who have the condition.

Lifestyle Techniques

Changing one's lifestyle can have a big impact on how osteoarthritis (OA) is managed and how healthy joints are overall. The following lifestyle suggestions are for people who have osteoarthritis:

Sustain a Healthy Weight:

The key to lessening the strain on weight-bearing joints like the knees and hips is to reach and maintain a healthy weight. Losing weight can help with osteoarthritis symptoms and delay the disease's progression.

Exercise on a Regular Basis:

Walking, swimming, and cycling are examples of low-impact workouts that help strengthen muscles, lessen pain, and increase joint flexibility. To create a customized workout program, speak with a physical therapist or healthcare professional.

Together-Friendly Activities:

Select joint-friendly exercises like stationary cycling, swimming, and water aerobics. These workouts strengthen the heart without putting undue strain on the joints.

Strengthening Exercise:

Incorporate workouts for strength training to develop and preserve muscle strength. Robust muscles stabilize the joints, lessening the strain on the cartilage.

Movement Range Exercises:

Exercises with mild range-of-motion should be done to keep joints flexible. To decrease stiffness and increase mobility, perform these exercises on a daily basis.

Collaborative Defense Strategies:

To reduce joint stress during regular tasks, educate yourself on joint protection strategies and put them into practice. Using assistive technology, practicing good body mechanics, and avoiding undue joint strain are a few examples of this.

A well-rounded diet

Eat a diet high in fruits, vegetables, whole grains, lean proteins, and balance to ensure optimal health. Antioxidants and omega-3 fatty acids are two examples of foods that may have anti-inflammatory qualities.

Maintain Hydration:

To keep joints well-hydrated throughout the day, make sure you drink enough water. Drinking enough water is crucial for healthy joints.

Warm and Chilled Treatment:

To relieve discomfort, apply heat or ice to the afflicted joints. While cold packs can lessen inflammation, warm compresses or heating pads can aid with muscle relaxation.

Control Your Stress:

Use stress-relieving methods including yoga, meditation, and deep breathing. Stress can worsen the symptoms of osteoarthritis and lead to muscle tightness.

Proper Posture:

To lessen the tension on the spine and joints, maintain proper posture. Additionally, ergonomic changes made at home and at work can promote improved joint health.

Fitting Footwear:

Put on cozy, arch-supporting shoes that are supportive. This is especially crucial for people whose knees, ankles, or feet are affected by osteoarthritis.

Restful Sleep:

Make sure you receive enough restful sleep. In addition to being beneficial for general health, getting enough sleep can help with pain perception and healing.

Steer clear of overexertion:

When engaging in activities, pace yourself to prevent overexertion. To avoid putting too much strain on your joints, take rests and pay attention to your body.

Frequent Medical Examinations:

Make an appointment for routine examinations with medical professionals to track the progression of osteoarthritis symptoms, evaluate joint function, and modify the treatment strategy as needed.

By implementing these lifestyle changes, osteoarthritis can be effectively managed and a healthier, more active lifestyle can be encouraged. It's critical that patients collaborate closely with their medical team to customize these tactics to meet their unique demands and take care of any issues or symptom changes.

Nutritional Aspects

Due to its ability to supply vital nutrients, maintain joint health, and possibly lower inflammation, diet is an important component of osteoarthritis (OA) management. Although there isn't a set "OA diet," people with osteoarthritis may benefit from the following dietary considerations:

The Fatty Acids Omega-3:

Consume foods high in omega-3 fatty acids, such as walnuts, flaxseeds, chia seeds, and fatty fish (salmon, mackerel, and sardines). Due to their anti-inflammatory qualities, omega-3s may be able to reduce stiffness and pain in the joints.

Rich in Antioxidants Foods:

Eat a range of foods high in antioxidants, such as vibrant fruits and vegetables (kale, spinach, cherries, and berries), as these may help lessen joint inflammation and oxidative stress.

Vitamin D and calcium:

Make sure you're getting enough calcium and vitamin D for strong bones. Good sources include dairy products, leafy greens, plant-based milk that has been fortified, and sunshine exposure.

Rich in Collagen Foods:

A protein called collagen helps maintain the health of cartilage and joints. Eat more collagen-rich items in your diet, including as fish and chicken skins, as well as bone broth.

Ginger and Turmeric:

Ginger and turmeric are both anti-inflammatory foods. Use these spices in your food or think about putting them in smoothies.

Green Tea:

Polyphenols found in green tea may have anti-inflammatory properties. It can be a helpful and hydrating drink for people who have osteoarthritis.

Good Fats:

Select foods like almonds, avocados, and olive oil that are high in healthful fats. These fats support the general health of joints and may have anti-inflammatory properties.

Sustain a Healthy Weight:

To assist in maintaining a healthy weight, adopt a diet that is portion-controlled and balanced. The symptoms of osteoarthritis are exacerbated by excess body weight because it puts more strain on weight-bearing joints.

Eat Fewer Processed Foods:

Eat fewer refined and processed foods because they may aggravate inflammation. Pick complete, unprocessed foods whenever you can.

CHAPTER THREE

Reduce the amount of added sugars:

Reduce the amount of food and drink that has added sugar. Consuming too much sugar can have a detrimental effect on general health and aggravate inflammation.

Maintain Hydration:

To keep joints well-hydrated throughout the day, make sure you drink enough water. Drinking enough water is crucial for healthy joints.

Restrict Red Meat:

Red and processed meats should be consumed in moderation since they may be linked to elevated inflammation. Select sources of lean protein such as fish, chicken, and plant-based proteins.

Supplemental glucosamine and chondroitin:

Some people with osteoarthritis might think about taking supplements containing chondroitin and glucosamine. Before beginning any new supplement regimen, speak with your doctor.

It's crucial to remember that everyone may react differently to dietary modifications. A customized eating plan based on your unique requirements, tastes, and medical circumstances can be created by consulting with a healthcare provider or a licensed dietitian. Furthermore, getting a wide range of nutrients that promote general health and joint function requires eating a well-balanced, diversified diet.

How to Handle Osteoarthritis

Osteoarthritis (OA) can be managed using a combination of self-management techniques, lifestyle modifications, and emotional health techniques. The following coping mechanisms can assist people in overcoming the difficulties associated with having osteoarthritis:

Knowledge and comprehension:

Find more about the causes of osteoarthritis and how it impacts the joints. People who are aware of the illness are better able to take an active role in their care and make wise decisions.

Self-Observation:

Maintain a record of your symptoms, degree of pain, and any environmental or dietary factors that may be linked to your osteoarthritis. Effective management of the condition can be aided by the knowledge provided.

Pain Reduction Methods:

Investigate other methods of treating pain, such as deep breathing exercises, heat or cold therapy, and relaxation techniques. By using these techniques, pain can be reduced and general comfort can be increased.

Collaborative Defense Strategies:

To reduce the amount of strain on the impacted joints during daily activities, learn and put these joint protection strategies into practice. Using assistive technology, practicing good body mechanics, and avoiding activities that worsen symptoms are a few examples of this.

Engaging in Exercise:

Regularly perform low-impact exercises to keep your muscles strong and your joints flexible. Create a personalized workout regimen with a physical therapist that fits your needs and preferences.

Controlling Weight:

In order to lessen the strain on weight-bearing joints, maintain a healthy weight. If required, losing weight can greatly reduce osteoarthritis symptoms and decrease the disease's progression.

Adaptive Technology:

To support joint function and lessen tension on afflicted areas, think about utilizing adaptive equipment like braces, splints, or assistive tools.

Comfortable Footwear:

Invest in supportive, cozy shoes that provide appropriate arch support. Proper footwear can have a good effect on joint health, particularly if you have osteoarthritis in your knees, ankles, or feet.

A well-rounded diet

Eat a healthy, well-balanced diet to promote general wellbeing. Antioxidants and omega-3 fatty acids are two examples of foods that may have anti-inflammatory properties.

Social Assistance:

Participate in support groups or share your experiences with friends and family to create a network of people who can help you. Making connections with people who have comparable difficulties might offer understanding and emotional support.

Support for Mental Health and Counseling:

If necessary, seek therapy or mental health assistance. Talking to a mental health professional can offer coping mechanisms and emotional support for those who live with chronic pain, which can have an influence on mental health.

Adjustments for Work and Home:

Make changes to your living and working spaces to promote joint health. This could entail altering daily routines, utilizing assistive technology, and making ergonomic adjustments.

Adaptability and Flexibility:

In your day-to-day tasks, embrace adaptation and flexibility. Pay attention to your body, pace yourself, and be prepared to adjust duties to suit your requirements.

Frequent Examinations:

Make an appointment for routine examinations with medical professionals to track the progression of osteoarthritis symptoms, evaluate joint function, and modify the treatment strategy as needed.

Osteoarthritis coping is a dynamic process that calls for constant self-management and teamwork with medical professionals. Despite the difficulties presented by osteoarthritis, people can improve their quality of life and continue to lead active, satisfying lives by combining a variety of tactics.

CONCLUSION

In conclusion, millions of people worldwide are greatly impacted by osteoarthritis, a prevalent degenerative joint illness. Although osteoarthritis cannot be cured, there are a number of ways to manage symptoms, strengthen joints, and improve general health.

Individuals are empowered to actively participate in their care through the comprehensive approach to managing osteoarthritis, which includes everything from exercise and lifestyle changes to pain management strategies and adaptable technologies. Developing a solid support system, getting help from medical specialists, and being aware of the condition all help people deal with osteoarthritis effectively.

Although osteoarthritis is a chronic condition, there is still hope for better results and a higher quality of life for individuals who live with it because to advancements in research, medications, and tailored care plans. People with osteoarthritis can traverse the path with resilience and continue to lead active and meaningful lives by adopting a proactive mentality, being informed, and putting customized methods into practice. A thorough and effective management of osteoarthritis is facilitated by frequent examinations, continuous self-monitoring, and a holistic approach to general health.

THE END